Guarding Against Syphilis

*The Definitive Handbook for Navigating
the Maze of Symptoms, Diagnosis,
Treatment and Recovery from the
Sneakiest STD*

(Things You Must Know)

By

Isabella White

About the Book

Syphilis earned its reputation as **"the great imitator"** for a good reason: its diverse symptoms and multiple stages can make it incredibly difficult to recognize and diagnose. This cunning sexually transmitted disease can seem to disappear for years only to re-emerge in its most devastating form if left untreated.

In *Guarding Against Syphilis,* you will find the most comprehensive, up-to-date guide to protecting yourself and your loved ones from this stealthy infection. Within these pages, leading medical experts provide authoritative information and practical strategies for every step of the syphilis journey, from dodging infection in the first place to seeking an accurate diagnosis, finding the most effective treatment, and learning what to expect on the road to recovery.

This definitive handbook dispels common myths and misconceptions about syphilis while arming you with the knowledge you need to avoid becoming one of the over 100,000 new cases diagnosed in the U.S. each year. Learn to recognize the distinctive rashes, sores, and flu-like symptoms of primary and secondary syphilis. Discover what to look for when the disease enters its latent "hiding" phase. Understand why routine STD testing is crucial for early detection. Get the facts to ensure you receive the right diagnosis.

From treatment options like penicillin and doxycycline to dealing with Jarisch-Herxheimer reactions, Guarding Against Syphilis lays out specialized regimens for every patient scenario. You will also find invaluable advice for supporting recovery through follow-up exams, addressing stigma, and preventing reinfection.

Do not leave yourself vulnerable to the ravages of **"the great pretender."** Arm yourself with the definitive guide to outsmarting syphilis at every turn. Let *Guarding Against Syphilis* chart your course to healthier relationships, peace of mind, and staying syphilis-free for life!

Introduction

What is Syphilis and Why is it Called the Sneakiest STD?

Syphilis is a bacterial infection that can be transmitted through sexual contact, blood transfusion, or from mother to child during pregnancy or birth. Syphilis can cause serious health problems if left untreated, such as damage to the heart, brain, or other organs.

Syphilis is often called the sneakiest STD because it can have no symptoms or very mild ones that are easy to miss or confuse with other diseases. Syphilis can also lie dormant for years without causing any problems but then reappear and cause complications. Syphilis can mimic the symptoms of many other conditions, such as rashes, ulcers, fever, hair loss, and neurological problems. This makes it difficult to diagnose and treat syphilis without proper testing and medical care.

How Common is Syphilis, and Who is at Risk?

Syphilis is a common and serious sexually transmitted infection (STI) that can affect anyone who is sexually active. According to the World Health Organization (WHO), about 7.1 million adults between 15 and 49 years old acquired syphilis in 2020. Syphilis is especially prevalent among key populations, such as gay men and other men who have sex with men (MSM), who are disproportionately affected by the disease.

Some factors that increase the risk of getting syphilis include:

- Having multiple sexual partners or changing partners frequently
- Having unprotected sex (oral, vaginal, or anal) without using condoms or dental dams
- Having sex under the influence of alcohol or drugs
- Having a history of other STIs or HIV

- Having sex with someone who has syphilis or other STIs
- Receiving an unscreened blood transfusion
- Being pregnant or giving birth to a child with syphilis

Syphilis can be prevented by practicing safe sex, getting tested regularly, and seeking treatment as soon as possible if infected. Syphilis can be cured with antibiotics, but early diagnosis and treatment are essential to avoid complications and transmission.

What are the Main Goals of this Book, and How Do You Use it?

The main goals of this book are to:

- Provide clear and concise information about syphilis, its causes, symptoms, stages, diagnosis, treatment, and prevention.
- Offer holistic and effective strategies to cope with and overcome syphilis, such as lifestyle changes, emotional support, and alternative therapies.

- Empower you to take charge of your health and well-being and to protect yourself and your loved ones from this infection.
- Educate you about the risks and challenges of syphilis and how to deal with them.
- Inspire you to live a healthier and happier life despite having syphilis or being affected by it.

This book is designed to be a comprehensive and practical guide you can use at any stage of your journey with syphilis. You can read it from cover to cover or skip to the chapters or sections that are most relevant to you. You can also use it as a reference book to look up specific topics or questions that you may have.

This book is not intended to replace professional medical advice or care. It is meant to supplement and complement the services and support you receive from your doctor, nurse, or other health care provider. You should always consult your doctor before making any decisions or changes regarding your health or treatment. You should also follow the instructions and recommendations your doctor gives you and report any symptoms or side effects you may experience.

By reading this book, you will gain valuable knowledge and insights that will help you guard against syphilis and live a healthier and happier life. You will also join a community of people who share your experiences and challenges and support and encourage you. This book will be a valuable and helpful resource for you, and you will enjoy reading it as much as I enjoyed writing it.

Table of Contents

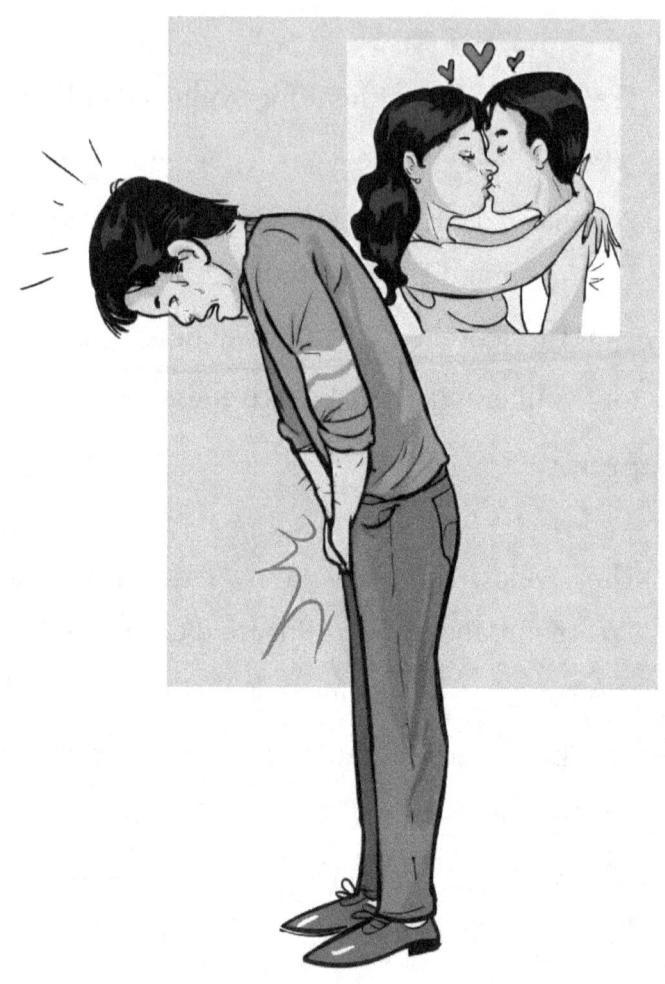

Chapter 1

Recognizing the Symptoms of Syphilis

The Four Stages of Syphilis and Their Signs and Complications

Syphilis is a bacterial infection that can be transmitted through sexual contact, blood transfusion, or from mother to child during pregnancy or birth. Syphilis can cause serious health problems if left untreated, such as damage to the heart, brain, or other organs.

Syphilis develops in four stages, each with its own set of symptoms and complications. The stages are:

- **Primary syphilis:** This is the first stage, which usually begins about three weeks after exposure to the bacteria. The main symptom is a small, painless sore called a chancre, which appears at the site of infection (such as the genitals, rectum, or mouth). The chancre heals within 3 to 6 weeks, but the infection remains in the body.

- **Secondary syphilis:** This is the second stage, which usually occurs a few weeks to months after the chancre heals. The main symptom is a rash that often covers the whole body, especially the palms of the hands and the soles of the feet. Other symptoms, such as fever, swollen lymph nodes, a sore throat, hair loss, and fatigue, may accompany the rash. These symptoms may come and go for months or years, but the infection remains in the body.

- **Latent syphilis:** This is the third stage, which occurs when the symptoms of secondary syphilis disappear. This stage can last for years or even decades, without any signs or symptoms of the infection. However, the bacteria are still alive in the body and can cause damage to the organs or reactivate at any time.

- **Tertiary syphilis:** This is the fourth and final stage, which occurs when the infection becomes active again after a long period of latency. This stage can cause serious and life-threatening complications, such as heart disease, stroke, brain damage, nerve damage, blindness, deafness, paralysis, and death. This stage can occur anytime after the initial infection but usually happens 10 to 30 years later.

The symptoms and complications of syphilis can vary from person to person, depending on the stage of the infection, the duration of the infection, the immune system of the person, and the treatment received. Some people may have mild or no symptoms, while others may have severe or fatal symptoms. Some people may skip or repeat some stages, while others may progress through all the stages.

The only way to know for sure if you have syphilis is to get tested by a healthcare provider. Blood tests, fluid tests, or a physical examination can diagnose syphilis. Syphilis can be cured with antibiotics, but early diagnosis and treatment are essential to prevent complications and transmission.

How to Recognize Early Symptoms and Avoid Misdiagnosis

Recognizing the early symptoms of syphilis and avoiding misdiagnosis are important steps to prevent the infection from progressing and causing complications. Here are some tips to help you:

- Be aware of the first sign of syphilis, which is a small, painless sore called a chancre that appears at the site of infection, usually the genitals, rectum, or mouth. The sore may be hidden or hard to see, so you should check yourself regularly and look for unusual bumps or lesions. The sore usually develops about three weeks after exposure to the bacteria, but it can range from 10 to 90 days.

- If you notice a sore, get tested for syphilis as soon as possible. A blood or fluid test from the sore can confirm the diagnosis. Please do not rely on self-diagnosis or home testing kits, as they may not be accurate or reliable.

- If you have a sore, avoid sexual contact until you get tested and treated. Syphilis is highly contagious and can spread through direct contact with the sore. You should also inform your sexual partners that you have a sore and that they should get tested, too.
- If you have a negative test result but still have symptoms or have been exposed to someone with syphilis, you should get tested again after a few weeks. Sometimes, the test may not detect the infection in the early stages or give a false negative result. You should also get tested for other sexually transmitted infections (STIs), as syphilis can increase the risk of getting or transmitting other STIs.
- If you have a positive test result, you should start treatment immediately. Syphilis can be cured with antibiotics, usually penicillin. Follow the instructions and recommendations of your healthcare provider and complete the full course of treatment. You should also get tested again after treatment to ensure the infection is gone.

- If you have no symptoms but have been exposed to someone with syphilis, you should also get tested and treated. Syphilis can have no symptoms or very mild ones that are easy to miss or confuse with other diseases. Syphilis can also lie dormant for years without causing any problems but then reappear and cause complications. Therefore, it is better to be safe than sorry and get tested and treated immediately.

By recognizing the early symptoms of syphilis and avoiding misdiagnosis, you can prevent the infection from advancing and harming your health.

How to Monitor your Symptoms and When to Seek Medical Attention

Monitoring your symptoms and seeking medical attention when needed are crucial steps to ensure your recovery from syphilis and prevent complications. Here are some tips to help you:

- Keep track of your symptoms and how they change over time. You can use a diary, a calendar, or an app to record your symptoms, such as the date, location, appearance, and severity of any sores, rashes, or other signs. You can also take pictures of your symptoms to show your healthcare provider.

- Follow up with your health care provider regularly, as they recommend. You will need to get tested for syphilis again after treatment to make sure the infection is gone. You may also need to get tested for other sexually transmitted infections (STIs), as syphilis can increase the risk of getting or transmitting other STIs.
- Seek medical attention immediately if you experience any of the following symptoms, as they may indicate serious complications of syphilis:
  o Severe headache, stiff neck, or confusion.
  o Vision problems, such as blurred vision, double vision, or blindness
  o Hearing problems, such as ringing in the ears, deafness, or balance issues
  o Numbness, tingling, or weakness in any part of the body

- o Difficulty speaking, swallowing, or moving
- o Chest pain, shortness of breath, or palpitations
- o Abdominal pain, swelling, or jaundice
- o Skin ulcers, nodules, or tumors
- Seek medical attention as soon as possible if you experience any of the following symptoms, as they may indicate a recurrence or reinfection of syphilis:
  - o A new or persistent sore on the skin or mucous membranes, especially on the genitals, rectum, or mouth
  - o A new or persistent rash, especially on the palms of the hands and the soles of the feet
  - o Fever, swollen lymph nodes, sore throat, or fatigue
  - o Hair loss, weight loss, or muscle aches

By monitoring your symptoms and seeking medical attention when needed, you can ensure your recovery from syphilis and prevent complications.

Chapter 2

The Diagnosis of Syphilis

The Different Types of Tests for Syphilis and How They Work

To diagnose syphilis, your health care provider may use different types of tests that look for either the bacteria that causes syphilis or the antibodies that your immune system produces to fight the infection. The type of test you need depends on your symptoms, medical history, and risk factors. Here are some of the common tests for syphilis and how they work:

- **Screening tests:** These are blood tests that check for antibodies linked to a syphilis infection. However, these antibodies may also be present due to other conditions, such as autoimmune diseases, infections, or vaccinations. Therefore, these tests could be more specific and give false-positive results. Screening tests for syphilis include the following:

o **Rapid plasma reagin (RPR):** This test measures the level of an antibody called reagin, which reacts with a substance called cardiolipin. The cells damaged by syphilis bacteria release cardiolipin. The higher the level of reagin, the more likely you are to have syphilis. However, reagin can also be produced by other diseases or conditions, such as lupus, malaria, or pregnancy.

o **Venereal Disease Research Laboratory (VDRL):** This test is similar to the RPR test, but it can also be done on spinal fluid, which is the fluid that surrounds the brain and spinal cord. This test can help diagnose neurosyphilis, which is a complication of syphilis that affects the nervous system. However, this test can also give false positive results due to other causes of inflammation in the spinal fluid, such as meningitis, tuberculosis, or cancer.

- **Confirmatory tests:** These are tests that check for antibodies that are specific to syphilis bacteria. When your immune system encounters syphilis bacteria, it produces antibodies that remain in your blood for a long time, even after treatment. Therefore, these tests are more accurate and reliable than screening tests but cannot distinguish between a current or past infection. Confirmatory tests for syphilis include the following:

  o *Treponema pallidum particle agglutination assay (TP-PA):* This test uses red blood cells coated with syphilis bacteria to detect the presence of syphilis antibodies in your blood. If you have syphilis antibodies, they will bind to the coated red blood cells and cause them to clump together. This clumping can be seen under a microscope.

  o *Fluorescent treponemal antibody absorption (FTA-ABS) test:* This test uses a fluorescent dye to label syphilis bacteria and then mixes them with your blood sample. If you have syphilis antibodies, they will bind to the labeled bacteria and make them glow under a special light. This test can also be done on spinal fluid to diagnose neurosyphilis.

o **Other tests:** Similar methods are used to detect syphilis antibodies, such as micro hemagglutination assays for T. pallidum antibodies (MHA-TP), T. pallidum hemagglutination assays (TPHA), T. pallidum enzyme immunoassays (TP-EIA), and chemiluminescence immunoassays (CLIA). These tests may vary in sensitivity and specificity and may not be available in all laboratories.

• **Direct tests:** These tests look for the actual Syphilis bacteria instead of antibodies. These tests are used less often because they require a sample of fluid or tissue from a sore or lesion, which may not be present or accessible in some cases. These tests are also more complex and expensive and can only be done in specialized labs. Direct tests for syphilis include:

- *Darkfield microscopy:* This test uses a special microscope to examine a fluid sample from a sore or lesion. The microscope has a dark background and a bright light illuminating the sample. If syphilis bacteria are present, they will appear as thin, spiral-shaped organisms that move around. This test can only be done on fresh samples, and it may not be reliable if other bacteria contaminate the sample.
- *Polymerase chain reaction (PCR):* This test uses a technique called PCR to amplify and detect the DNA of syphilis bacteria in a sample of fluid or tissue from a sore or lesion. This test is susceptible and specific, but it may need to be widely available or standardized.

These are the different types of tests for syphilis and how they work. Your healthcare provider will decide which test or combination is best for you based on your symptoms, medical history, and risk factors. If you test positive for syphilis, you will need to start treatment as soon as possible to prevent complications and transmission. If you test negative for syphilis but you still have symptoms or have been exposed to someone with syphilis, you may need to get tested again after a few weeks, as some tests may not detect the infection in the early stages.

The Pros and Cons of Each Test and How to Choose the Best One for You

Each test for syphilis has its pros and cons, and the best one for you depends on your situation and preferences. Here are some factors to consider when choosing a test for syphilis:

- **Accuracy:** Some tests are more sensitive and specific than others, meaning they are more likely to detect the infection and less likely to give false positive or negative results. Generally, confirmatory tests and direct tests are more accurate than screening tests, but they may only be available or affordable in some settings.

- **Speed:** Some tests are faster and easier to perform than others, meaning they can give you results sooner and with less hassle. Generally, screening and direct tests are faster and simpler than confirmatory tests but may only be conclusive or definitive in some cases.

- **Cost:** Some tests are more expensive and require more resources than others, meaning they may not be accessible or affordable for everyone. Generally, confirmatory tests and direct tests are costlier and complex than screening tests, but they may be more reliable and informative in the long run.

- **Availability:** Certain medical tests are more commonly accessible and have standard procedures compared to others. This means they can be easily located and compared across different healthcare settings. Screening and confirmatory tests are typically more standardized and widely available than direct tests. However, ensuring that the selected tests are suitable for the situation and sufficient to provide accurate results is important.

To choose the best test for you, you should consult your healthcare provider, who can advise you based on your symptoms, medical history, and risk factors. You should also consider your personal preferences, such as how quickly you want to know your status, how much you are willing to pay, and how comfortable you are with different tests. You should also be aware of the limitations and implications of each test and be prepared to follow up with further testing or treatment if needed.

How to Prepare for the Test and What to Expect from the Results

To prepare for the test and what to expect from the results, here are some tips to help you:

- Depending on the type of test you need, you may have to provide a blood, fluid, or tissue sample. You may need to fast for blood tests for a few hours before the test. For fluid tests, you may need to avoid urinating for an hour before the test. For tissue tests, you may need to have a small piece of skin or mucous membrane removed from a sore or lesion.

- The test results may take a few minutes to a few days to come back, depending on the type of test and the laboratory. Ask your healthcare provider when and how you will receive your results and if you need to make a follow-up appointment.

- The test results may be reported as positive, negative, or indeterminate. A positive result means that you have syphilis or that you had it in the past. A negative result means that you do not have syphilis or that you have it in the early stages. An indeterminate result means that the test is inconclusive or has a discrepancy between different tests.

- The test results may also include a number indicating the titer of antibodies in your blood. This number may change over time, depending on the stage of the infection and the treatment received. A higher number usually means a more active or recent infection, while a lower number usually means a less active or older infection. However, this number is only sometimes reliable or consistent and may vary from person to person and from lab to lab.

- The test results may not be definitive or final and may need to be confirmed or repeated with another test. This is because some tests could be more specific and sensitive, and they may give false positive or negative results. You should consult your health care provider to interpret your test results and decide on the next steps.

Preparing for the test and knowing what to expect from the results can make the process easier and more accurate.

Chapter 3

The Treatment of Syphilis

The Standard Treatment for Syphilis and How it Works

The standard treatment for syphilis is the antibiotic penicillin, which can cure the infection and prevent further damage, but it cannot repair damage already done. Penicillin works by killing the bacteria that causes syphilis, called Treponema pallidum.

The type and dose of penicillin depend on the stage of syphilis and the presence of any complications. Generally, the treatment for syphilis is as follows:

- **Primary, secondary, or early latent syphilis:** A single injection of long-acting benzathine penicillin G is usually enough to cure the infection. This stage includes the first year of infection, when symptoms such as sores, rashes, or fever may occur.

- **Late latent syphilis or syphilis of unknown duration**: Three doses of long-acting benzathine penicillin G at weekly intervals are recommended to cure the infection. This stage includes infections that have lasted longer than a year or when the duration of the infection is unclear. Symptoms may not be present, but the infection can still cause damage to the organs.

- **Tertiary syphilis or neurosyphilis:** High doses of intravenous penicillin G or intramuscular procaine penicillin with oral probenecid for 10 to 14 days are required to treat the infection. This stage includes infections that have become active again after a long period of latency and that have caused severe and life-threatening complications, such as heart disease, stroke, brain damage, nerve damage, blindness, deafness, paralysis, and death.

People allergic to penicillin may be given other antibiotics, such as doxycycline, tetracycline, ceftriaxone, or azithromycin. However, these alternatives may not be as effective or safe as penicillin, especially for pregnant people or people with HIV. People allergic to penicillin may also undergo desensitization, which involves gradually taking small amounts of penicillin until the body can tolerate it. This process is done by a specialist called an allergist or an immunologist.

People who are treated for syphilis should follow the instructions and recommendations of their healthcare provider and complete the full course of treatment. They should also get tested after treatment to ensure the infection is gone. They should avoid sexual contact with new partners until the treatment is finished and any sores are completely healed. They should also inform their sexual partners that they have syphilis so they can get tested and treated if needed.

By getting the standard treatment for syphilis, people can prevent the infection from progressing and causing complications.

Possible Side Effects and Complications of the Treatment and How to Manage Them

The treatment for syphilis is usually effective and safe, but it may cause some side effects and complications in some people. Here are some of the possible side effects and complications of the treatment and how to manage them:

- **Allergic reaction:** Some people may be allergic to penicillin or other antibiotics used to treat syphilis. Symptoms of an allergic reaction may include rash, itching, swelling, difficulty breathing, or anaphylaxis (a severe and life-threatening reaction). If you have a history of penicillin allergies, you should tell your healthcare provider before starting treatment. You may need to undergo desensitization, which involves gradually taking small amounts of penicillin until the body can tolerate it. This process is done by a specialist called an allergist or an immunologist. If you develop an allergic reaction during or after treatment, you should seek medical attention immediately. You may need to take antihistamines, steroids, or epinephrine to treat the reaction.

- **Jarisch-Herxheimer reaction:** This is a reaction that occurs when the syphilis bacteria die and release toxins into the blood. Symptoms of this reaction may include fever, headache, joint or muscle pain, nausea, and chills. This reaction usually happens within the first 24 hours of treatment and may last for a few hours or days. It is not an allergic reaction and does not mean the treatment is not working. You should drink plenty of fluids, take painkillers, and rest to manage this reaction. You should also inform your healthcare provider if you experience this reaction, as they may need to monitor your condition.

- **Pregnancy complications:** If you are pregnant and have syphilis, you may need to take higher doses of penicillin or other antibiotics to treat the infection and prevent it from passing on to your baby. However, these antibiotics may cause you or your baby side effects, such as nausea, diarrhea, or yeast infections. You should follow the instructions and recommendations of your healthcare provider and report any symptoms or side effects you experience. You should also get regular prenatal checkups and tests to monitor your health and your baby's health.

- **Treatment failure or reinfection:** In rare cases, the treatment for syphilis may fail to cure the infection or prevent it from coming back. This may happen if you do not complete the full course of treatment, if you have a resistant strain of syphilis bacteria, or if you get reinfected by a new or untreated partner. To prevent treatment failure or reinfection, you should follow the instructions and recommendations of your healthcare provider and complete the full course of treatment. You should also get tested again after treatment to ensure the infection is gone. You should avoid sexual contact with new partners until the treatment is finished and any sores are completely healed. You should also inform your sexual partners that you have syphilis so they can get tested and treated if needed.

By being aware of the possible side effects and complications of the treatment and how to manage them, you can improve your recovery from syphilis and prevent further damage.

The Alternative and Complementary Therapies for Syphilis and Their Effectiveness

Besides the standard treatment of antibiotics, some people may seek alternative and complementary therapies for syphilis. These therapies are not meant to replace conventional medicine but to supplement and enhance it. However, the evidence for the effectiveness and safety of these therapies is limited or lacking, and they may have side effects or interactions with other medications.

Therefore, you should always consult with your healthcare provider before trying any alternative or complementary therapy for syphilis. Here are some of the common alternative and complementary therapies for syphilis and their effectiveness:

- **Herbal remedies:** Some herbs may have antibacterial, anti-inflammatory, or immune-boosting properties that may help fight syphilis or ease its symptoms. However, there is not enough scientific research to support the use of these herbs for syphilis, and they may have adverse effects or interactions with other drugs. Some of the herbs that may be beneficial for syphilis include echinacea, garlic, and sarsaparilla.

- **Homeopathy:** Homeopathy is a system of medicine that uses highly diluted substances to stimulate the body's natural healing response. Homeopathy claims to treat syphilis by addressing its underlying causes and constitutional factors. However, there is no scientific evidence to support the effectiveness or safety of homeopathy for syphilis, and it may delay or interfere with conventional treatment. Some of the homeopathic remedies that may be used for syphilis include Mercurius, Aurum, and Syphilis.

- **Acupuncture:** Acupuncture is a technique that involves inserting thin needles into specific points on the body to balance the flow of energy, or qi. Acupuncture may help relieve pain, inflammation, or stress associated with syphilis or its treatment. However, there is not enough scientific evidence to support the effectiveness or safety of acupuncture for syphilis, and it may pose risks of infection or bleeding. Acupuncture should only be performed by a qualified and licensed practitioner.

- **Aromatherapy:** Aromatherapy is the use of essential oils extracted from plants to enhance physical, mental, or emotional well-being. Aromatherapy may help improve mood, relaxation, or sleep quality for people with syphilis or its treatment. However, there is not enough scientific evidence to support the effectiveness or safety of aromatherapy for syphilis, and it may cause allergic reactions or interactions with other drugs. Aromatherapy should only be used with caution and under the guidance of a professional. Some essential oils that may be helpful for syphilis include lavender, tea tree, and rosemary.

These are the alternative and complementary therapies for syphilis and their effectiveness. You should always consult with your healthcare provider before trying any of these therapies, and you should only stop or change your conventional treatment with their approval. You should also inform your healthcare provider of any alternative or complementary therapies you use or plan to use, as they may affect your diagnosis, treatment, or outcome.

Chapter 4

The Recovery from Syphilis

The Follow-Up Care and Tests After the Treatment and How to Ensure a Complete Cure

The recovery from syphilis depends on the stage and severity of the infection, the effectiveness and timeliness of the treatment, and the presence of any complications or co-infections. To ensure a full recovery and prevent further damage, following the recommended follow-up care and testing from your healthcare provider is crucial.

Here are some of the follow-up care and tests after the treatment and how to ensure a complete cure:

- **Follow-up blood tests and exams:** You will need regular blood tests and exams to monitor your response to the treatment and check for any signs of recurrence or reinfection. The frequency and duration of the follow-up tests depend on the stage and clinical manifestations of syphilis, as well as your risk factors and medical history. Generally, the follow-up tests are done between 6 and 12 months after treatment and annually if needed. The follow-up tests may include:
  - *Nontreponemal tests:* These are screening tests that measure the level of antibodies linked to a syphilis infection, such as the rapid plasma reagin (RPR) or the venereal disease research laboratory (VDRL) tests. These tests are not specific and may give false-positive results due to other conditions. However, they can show the progress of the treatment by comparing the titers or numbers of the tests over time. A fourfold decrease in the titer (e.g., from

1:32 to 1:8) within 6 to 12 months after treatment indicates a successful treatment. A stable or increasing titer may indicate a treatment failure or a reinfection.

- o **Treponemal tests:** These are confirmatory tests that detect antibodies that are specific to syphilis bacteria, such as the treponema pallidum particle agglutination assay (TP-PA) or the fluorescent treponemal antibody absorption (FTA-ABS) test. These tests are more accurate and reliable than nontreponemal tests but cannot distinguish between a current or past infection. These tests usually remain positive for life, even after treatment. However, some people may experience a seroreversion or a negative result after successful treatment, especially if they were treated in the early stages of syphilis.
- o **Physical examination:** You will also need to have a physical examination to

look for any signs or symptoms of syphilis, such as sores, rashes, or lesions. You should also report any changes or concerns to your healthcare provider, such as fever, headache, joint or muscle pain, vision or hearing problems, or neurological issues.

- **Spinal fluid examination:** If you have signs or symptoms of neurosyphilis, which is a complication of syphilis that affects the nervous system, you will need to have a spinal fluid examination to diagnose and treat the infection. This involves taking a sample of the fluid surrounding the brain and spinal cord, called cerebrospinal fluid (CSF), by inserting a needle between two bones in the back. This procedure is called a lumbar puncture or a spinal tap. The CSF sample is tested for syphilis bacteria, antibodies, or inflammation.

- **Treatment completion and adherence:** You should complete the full course of treatment prescribed by your healthcare provider and follow their instructions and recommendations. You should not stop or change your treatment without their approval, and you should report any side effects or reactions that you experience. You should also avoid sexual contact with new partners until the treatment is finished and any sores are completely healed. You should also inform your sexual partners that you have syphilis so they can get tested and treated if needed.

By following the follow-up care and tests after the treatment and ensuring a complete cure, you can recover from syphilis and prevent further damage. You can also protect yourself and your loved ones from this infection by practicing safe sex, getting tested regularly, and seeking treatment as soon as possible.

The Long-Term Effects and Complications of Syphilis and How to Prevent Them

Syphilis is a severe infection that can cause long-term effects and complications if left untreated or treated too late. Some of the possible long-term effects and complications of syphilis are:

- **Neurosyphilis:** This is a condition that affects the brain and nervous system. It can cause symptoms such as headaches, stiff necks, confusion, vision problems, hearing problems, numbness, weakness, difficulty speaking, swallowing, or moving, and dementia. Neurosyphilis can occur at any stage of syphilis, but it is more common in the late stage. It can be diagnosed by a spinal fluid examination and treated with high doses of intravenous penicillin or other antibiotics.

- **Cardiovascular syphilis:** This is a condition that affects the heart and blood vessels. It can cause problems such as inflammation of the aorta (the main artery that carries blood from the heart), aneurysms (a bulge or rupture in the wall of an artery), heart valve damage, heart failure, and chest pain. Cardiovascular syphilis usually occurs in the late stage of syphilis, 10 to 30 years after the initial infection. It can be diagnosed by physical examination, blood tests, and imaging tests and treated with antibiotics and surgery.

- **Gummatous syphilis:** This condition causes soft, noncancerous growths called gummas to form in various organs, such as the skin, bones, liver, and lungs. Gummas can cause pain, swelling, ulcers, and tissue damage. Gummatous syphilis usually occurs in the late stage of syphilis, 3–10 years after the initial infection. It can be diagnosed by biopsy and treated with antibiotics and surgery.

- **Congenital syphilis:** This is a condition that occurs when a pregnant person with syphilis passes the infection to their baby during pregnancy or childbirth. It can cause severe problems for the baby, such as miscarriage, stillbirth, premature birth, low birth weight, congenital disabilities, and death. Congenital syphilis can be prevented by testing and treating the pregnant person and their partner before or during pregnancy. It can be diagnosed by blood tests and a physical examination of the baby and treated with antibiotics.

- **HIV co-infection:** Having syphilis can increase the risk of getting or transmitting HIV, the virus that causes AIDS. This is because syphilis sores can make it easier for HIV to enter or leave the body during sexual contact. Also, having syphilis can weaken the immune system and make it harder to fight HIV. Having HIV can also make syphilis harder to diagnose and treat and increase the chances of complications. HIV co-infection can be prevented by practicing safe sex, getting tested regularly, and taking antiretroviral therapy if needed.

The best way to prevent the long-term effects and complications of syphilis is to avoid getting infected in the first place. This can be done by practicing safe sex, using condoms or dental dams during any sexual contact, and avoiding multiple or unknown sexual partners. It is also important to get tested for syphilis and other sexually transmitted infections (STIs) regularly, especially if you have symptoms or risk factors.

Lifestyle Changes and Habits to Boost Your Immune System and Prevent Reinfection

Besides getting the proper treatment for syphilis, you can also make some lifestyle changes and habits to boost your immune system and prevent reinfection.

Here are some of the lifestyle changes and habits that may help you:

- Eat a balanced and nutritious diet with plenty of fruits, vegetables, whole grains, lean proteins, and healthy fats. These foods can provide the vitamins, minerals, antioxidants, and other nutrients your body needs to fight infections and heal wounds. Some foods that may be especially beneficial for syphilis include garlic, onions, carrots, cauliflower, spinach, walnuts, almonds, pumpkin seeds, blue fish, eggs, and rice.

- Avoid foods that may worsen your symptoms or interfere with your treatment, such as sour buttermilk, heavy meals, alcohol, caffeine, sugar, and processed foods. These foods can lower your immunity, increase inflammation, or affect the absorption or effectiveness of your antibiotics.

- Drink fluids, especially water, to stay hydrated, flush out toxins, and prevent dehydration. Dehydration can cause headaches, fatigue, dry skin, and kidney problems. You should aim for at least eight glasses of water daily, or more if you are active, sick, or in a hot climate.

- Exercise regularly but moderately to improve blood circulation, oxygen delivery, muscle strength, and mood. Exercise can also help you manage stress, weakening your immune system and making you more susceptible to infections. However, you should not overdo it; too much or too intense exercise can have the opposite effect and lower your immunity. You should aim for at least 150 minutes of moderate aerobic activity, 75 minutes of vigorous aerobic activity a week, or a combination of both. You should also include some strength training and flexibility exercises in your routine.

- Get enough sleep and rest to allow your body and mind to recover and heal. Sleep is essential for your immune system, as it helps produce and regulate the cells and molecules that fight infections. Lack of sleep can impair your immunity, increase inflammation, and make you more prone to illnesses. You should aim for at least seven to nine hours of quality sleep a night and avoid distractions, stimulants, and interruptions that may disrupt your sleep. You should also take some time to relax and unwind during the day and avoid overwork and burnout.

- Quit smoking and avoid exposure to secondhand smoke, as smoking can damage your lungs, blood vessels, and immune system. Smoking can also increase your risk of complications from syphilis, such as cardiovascular disease, stroke, and cancer. Smoking can also make it harder for your antibiotics to work and increase the chances of treatment failure or reinfection. If you smoke, you should seek help to quit as soon as possible and avoid places or situations where you may be exposed to smoke.

- Practice safe sex and avoid multiple or unknown sexual partners, as syphilis is a sexually transmitted infection that can spread through oral, vaginal, or anal sex. You should use a condom or a dental dam every time you have sex and check yourself and your partner for any signs or symptoms of syphilis, such as sores, rashes, or lesions. You should also get tested for syphilis and other sexually transmitted infections (STIs) regularly, especially if you have symptoms or risk factors. If you test positive for syphilis, you should inform your sexual partners so they can get tested and treated if needed. You should also abstain from sexual contact until your treatment is finished and any sores are completely healed.

By making these lifestyle changes and habits, you can boost your immune system and prevent the reinfection of syphilis.

Conclusion

This book has provided you with clear and concise information about syphilis. This bacterial infection can be transmitted through sexual contact, blood transfusion, or from mother to child during pregnancy or birth. Syphilis can cause serious health problems if left untreated, such as damage to the heart, brain, or other organs.

Syphilis is often called the sneakiest STD because it can have no symptoms or very mild ones that are easy to miss or confuse with other diseases. Syphilis can also lie dormant for years without causing any problems but then reappear and cause complications.

In this book, you have learned about the following topics:

- The causes, symptoms, stages, diagnosis, treatment, and prevention of syphilis

- The holistic and effective strategies to cope with and overcome syphilis, such as lifestyle changes, emotional support, and alternative therapies
- The follow-up care and tests after the treatment and how to ensure a complete cure
- The long-term effects and complications of syphilis and how to prevent them
- Lifestyle changes and habits to boost your immune system and prevent reinfection

A Call to Action and Encouragement for The Readers to Take Charge of Their Health

Now that you have reached the end of this book, you may be wondering what to do next. How can you apply your knowledge to your situation and health? How can you make the most of the information and resources you gained from this book?

The answer is simple: take action. Do not let syphilis control your life or define who you are. You have the power and the responsibility to take charge of your health and well-being and to protect yourself and your loved ones from this infection. You have the tools and the support to cope with and overcome syphilis and to live a healthier and happier life.

Here are some of the actions that you can take to guard against syphilis and improve your health:

- Get tested for syphilis and other sexually transmitted infections (STIs) regularly, especially if you have symptoms or risk factors. Early diagnosis and treatment are essential to prevent complications and transmission. You can find a testing site near you by visiting this website.

- Follow the treatment your health care provider prescribes and complete the full course of antibiotics. Do not stop or change your treatment without their approval, and report any side effects or reactions you experience. You should also get tested again after treatment to ensure the infection is gone.

- Inform your sexual partners that you have syphilis so they can get tested and treated if needed. You should also abstain from sexual contact until your treatment is finished and any sores are completely healed. You can find tips and resources on how to talk to your partner about syphilis by visiting this website.

- Practice safe sex and avoid multiple or unknown sexual partners. Use a condom or a dental dam every time you have sex, and check yourself and your partner for any signs or symptoms of syphilis, such as sores, rashes, or lesions. You can find more information and advice on how to prevent syphilis and other STIs by visiting this website.

- Make lifestyle changes and habits to boost your immune system and prevent reinfection. Eat a balanced and nutritious diet, drink plenty of fluids, exercise regularly, get enough sleep and rest, quit smoking, and avoid stress. You can also try alternative and complementary therapies, such as herbal remedies, homeopathy, acupuncture, or aromatherapy, to supplement and enhance your conventional treatment. However, you should always consult with your healthcare provider before trying any of these therapies, and you should only stop or change your conventional treatment with their approval.

- Seek emotional and social support from your family, friends, or other people who have syphilis or are affected by it. You are not alone; you can overcome this infection with the right information, treatment, and support. You can also join a support group, an online community, or a counseling service to share your experiences and challenges and to receive advice and encouragement. You can find some of the support options by visiting this website.

By taking these actions, you can guard against syphilis and improve your health. You can also protect yourself and your loved ones from this infection by practicing safe sex, getting tested regularly, and seeking treatment as soon as possible.

By reading this book, you have gained valuable knowledge and insights that will help you guard against syphilis and live a healthier and happier life. You have also joined a community of people who share your experiences and challenges and support and encourage you. I hope this book has been a useful resource for you and that you have enjoyed reading it as much as I have enjoyed writing it.

Thank you for choosing this book, and we wish you all the best in your journey with syphilis. Remember, you are not alone and can overcome this infection with the right information, treatment, and support. Stay safe, stay healthy, and stay positive.

If you liked this book, please leave us a review and share it with your friends and family. Your feedback and support are greatly appreciated.

Thank you again, and take care.

Resources and References

If you want to learn more about syphilis or get support from other sources, you can check out the following resources and references:

- Syphilis - World Health Organization (WHO): This website provides key facts, overview, symptoms, diagnosis, treatment, and prevention of syphilis, as well as global statistics, publications, and news on syphilis.
- CDC – Syphilis Other Resources: This website offers various resources on syphilis, such as a call to action, success stories, webinars, guidance, and fact sheets.
- Syphilis infection - References | BMJ Best Practice US: This website lists the references used in the BMJ Best Practice topic on syphilis, which covers the causes, symptoms, stages, diagnosis, treatment, and prevention of

syphilis, as well as the holistic and effective strategies to cope with and overcome syphilis.

- [American Sexual Health Association (ASHA) - Syphilis]: This website provides information and advice on syphilis, such as what it is, how it is spread, how it is diagnosed and treated, and how it can be prevented. It also offers a helpline, a podcast, and a blog on syphilis and other sexual health topics.

- [Planned Parenthood - Syphilis]: This website provides information and services on syphilis, such as what it is, how it is transmitted, what the symptoms are, how it is tested and treated, and how it can be prevented. It also offers online chat, phone, and in-person support, as well as online tools to find a health center, book an appointment, or get birth control.